DRUGS USED WITH NEONATES AND DURING PREGNANCY

SECOND EDITION

DRUGS USED WITH NEONATES AND DURING PREGNANCY

SECOND EDITION

Ina Lee Stile, Pharm.D.

Thomas Hegyi, M.D.

I. Mark Hiatt, M.D.

Medical Economics Books
Oradell, NJ 07649

Library of Congress Cataloging in Publication Data

Stile, Ina Lee.
  Drugs used with neonates and during pregnancy.

  Includes index.
    1. Obstetrical pharmacology.   2. Infants (Newborn)—
Effect of drugs on.   3. Pediatric pharmacology.
I. Hegyi, Thomas.   II. Hiatt, I. Mark.   III. Title.
[DNLM: 1. Drug therapy—Adverse effects.   2. Fetus—
Drug effects.   3. Maternal-fetal exchange—Drug effects.
4. Pregnancy—Drug effects.   WQ 210 S856d]
RG131.S78   1983   615.5'8'0880542   83-7978
ISBN 0-87489-342-9

Cover design by Douglas Steel

ISBN 0-87489-342-9

Medical Economics Company Inc.
Oradell, New Jersey 07649

Printed in the United States of America

CONTENTS

PUBLISHER'S NOTES

The first edition of *Drugs Used With Neonates and During Pregnancy* was a 28-page booklet published in 1975. Its very wide distribution, requiring several printings, proved to us that it met a need among neonatologists, pediatricians, clinical pharmacists, and pediatric nurses.

In time, it became apparent that it was necessary to publish a new edition, greatly expanded and updated, to help these professionals face the challenges and changes of peri- and neonatal drug therapy.

The authors of this manual have produced exactly what was needed for such a revision. The result of their work—virtually a wholly new book—is a comprehensive review of drugs used in the pregnant woman, the neonate, and the nursing mother. The authors have also included a section on nutritional requirements of neonates fed enterally or parenterally. And they have supplied authoritative references for all the recommendations they make in the book.

Ina Lee Stile, Pharm.D., is assistant professor of clinical pharmacy, Rutgers University College of Pharmacy, Busch Campus, Piscataway, N.J. She is also clinical pharmacist in pediatrics and neonatology at St. Peter's Medical Center, New Brunswick, N.J.

Thomas Hegyi, M.D., and I. Mark Hiatt, M.D., are co-directors, Division of Neonatal Medicine, St. Peter's Medical Center, and co-directors, Newborn Intensive Care Unit, Monmouth Medical Center, Monmouth, N.J. Both are also clinical associate professors in the Department of Pediatrics at the University of Medicine and Dentistry of New Jersey-Rutgers Medical School.

Drugs in Pregnancy

Effects on the fetus and neonate

Medication	First trimester	Second and third trimesters, labor, and delivery
ALCOHOL	Fetal alcohol [1,2,3] syndrome: Mental retardation, microcephaly, craniofacial abnormalities, intrauterine growth retardation, cardiac anomalies (usually atrial-septal defect), limb deformities, retardation	Increased risk of [4] spontaneous abortions
ANALGESICS Narcotics		Central nervous system and respiratory depression; withdrawal syndrome following prolonged intrauterine exposure
Nonsteroidal anti-inflammatory agents		Abnormal platelet [4] function; closure of ductus arteriosus in utero, leading to persistent pulmonary hypertension in the newborn
Salicylates	Conflicting [3] data; may be associated with cleft palate and lip, hypospadias, and other congenital anomalies.	

Effects on the fetus and neonate

Medication	First trimester	Second and third trimesters, labor, and delivery
ANESTHESIA	Women working 3,5,6 in operating rooms exposed to inhalation agents may have increased incidence of spontaneous abortion and congenital malformations. Nitrous oxide inhibits activity of B_{12} and may be causative agent.	Central nervous 4,5 system depression, bradycardia, apnea, hypotonia, seizure

Note: Problems are more common after paracervical block. |
ANTICOAGULANTS	Fetal 4,7,8,9,10 warfarin syndrome: nasal hypoplasia, chondrodysplasia punctata	Fetal warfarin syn- 4,8 drome: optic atrophy, microcephaly, mental retardation, fetal and neonatal hemorrhage
	Note: Heparin is preferred for prevention of thromboembolic disease, except in patients with prosthetic valves, with whom benefits of warfarin outweigh risks. Heparin should be used in all patients who need anticoagulants during last three weeks of pregnancy.	
ANTICONVULSANTS	In general, infants 3 of women taking anticonvulsants have increased incidence of congenital malformations that include cleft palate and lip, cardiac anomalies, and skeletal defects.	Coagulation disturbances

Effects on the fetus and neonate

Medication	First trimester	Second and third trimesters, labor, and delivery
Carbamazepine (Tegretol)	No data	No data
Phenobarbital	Digital and [8,11] facial anomalies, congenital heart lesions	Hypocalcemia in the [12] newborn due to vitamin D deficiency; symptoms of drug withdrawal follow long-term exposure in utero. Administer vitamin K at birth.
Phenytoin (Dilantin)	Fetal hydantoin [9,11] syndrome— Craniofacial anomalies: low, broad nasal bridge; epicanthal folds; hypertelorism; ptosis; strabismus Limb defects: hypoplasia of the distal phalanges, fingerlike thumbs, alteration of the palmar crease Intrauterine growth retardation, mental retardation, congenital heart disease	Administer vitamin K at birth.
Primidone (Mysoline)	See phenobarbital.	See phenobarbital.

Medication	First trimester	Second and third trimesters, labor, and delivery
Trimethadione (Tridione)	V-shaped 9 eyebrows, low-set ears, palate abnormalities, developmental delay, speech disturbances, cardiac anomalies, intra-uterine growth retardation, ocular defects, simian creases, hypospadias, microcephaly	
Valproic acid (Depakene)	Risk of spina bifida	No data

ANTIMICROBIAL AGENTS		
Aminoglycosides	May cause auditory impairment due to damage to 4 eighth nerve. Streptomycin should not be used to treat tuberculosis during pregnancy, unless other first-line agents are ineffective.	
Chloramphenicol (Chloromycetin)		Risk of gray-baby syndrome if used during labor
Chloroquine (Aralen)	Conflicting data. May be associated with congenital 8 deafness. Nonetheless, it is drug of choice for treating malaria in pregnancy.	

Effects on the fetus and neonate

Medication	First trimester	Second and third trimesters, labor, and delivery
Pyrimethamine (Daraprim)	Theoretical risk of congenital abnormalities [3,8]	
Quinine	At high doses, [3] associated with hypoplasia of optic nerve and congenital deafness.	
Rifampin (Rifadin)		Risk of hypoprothrombinemia and bleeding; continues to be used in treating tuberculosis, if a third drug is needed.
Sulfonamides		Avoid use in G6PD deficient patients; theoretical risk of hyperbilirubinemia
Tetracycline	Tooth discoloration and enamel hypoplasia	
Trimethoprim	Theoretical risk of congenital abnormalities [3,8]	

Medication	First trimester	Second and third trimesters, labor, and delivery
CARDIOVASCULAR MEDICATIONS Magnesium sulfate		Side effects may occur [13] if used close to delivery: respiratory depression, hypotonia, convulsions, ileus.
Propranolol (Inderal)		Intrauterine growth retardation, bradycardia, hypoglycemia
Thiazide diuretics		Thrombocytopenia [3] (one case reported); theoretical risk of hypoglycemia
CYTOTOXIC AGENTS Alkylating agents	All cytotoxic agents [13] should be avoided if possible during first trimester Multiple congenital abnormalities	Intrauterine growth [8] retardation
Folate antagonists	Cleft palate, [3,7,12] cranial dysostoses, ear anomalies, skeletal defects, spontaneous abortion	

Effects on the fetus and neonate

Medication	First trimester	Second and third trimesters, labor, and delivery
DIPHENHYDRAMINE	May be associated *3,8* with cleft palate.	
ENDOCRINE THERAPY Androgens	Masculinization of female fetus, involving clitoral enlargement and fusion of labia with scrotal folds *8,14*	
Diethylstilbestrol	Vaginal *3,8* adenocarcinoma of female offspring, vaginal adenosis, uterine abnormalities, urogenital tract abnormalities in male offspring	
Estrogens	Masculinization of *8* female fetus	
Glucocorticoids	Risk of cleft *16* palate with high doses; intrauterine growth retardation	Monitor newborn *16* for adrenal insufficiency.

Medication	First trimester	Second and third trimesters, labor, and delivery
Oral contraceptives (combination of estrogen and progesterone)	Small risk [14,15] of congenital anomalies VACTREL syndrome: anomalies of the Vertebrae, Anus, Cardiovascular system, Trachea, Renal tract, Esophagus, and Limbs	
Oral hypoglycemic agents		Neonatal hypoglycemia [17]
Progesterone ethisterone norethisterone norethynodrel (Enovid)	Masculinization [14] of female fetus	
PSYCHOTHERAPY Chlordiazepoxide		Withdrawal syndrome [13] in the newborn following long-term exposure in utero

Effects on the fetus and neonate

Medication	First trimester	Second and third trimesters, labor, and delivery
Diazepam (Valium)	Conflicting data; [3] may be associated with an increased risk of cleft palate.	Withdrawal syndrome after long-term exposure in utero; administration prior to delivery may cause hypotonia, sedation, and poor feeding in the newborn. Doses > 30 mg during labor are associated with hypothermia and low Apgar score.
Haloperidol (Haldol)	Limb deformities [19] (two cases reported)	
Lithium	Cardiovascular [3] anomalies	Toxic levels may [4,20] produce hypotonia and cyanosis. Goiter, transient hypothyroidism, and nephrogenic diabetes insipidus have been reported.
Phenothiazines	Risk of limb deformities	Extrapyramidal reactions [4] in the newborn

Effects on the fetus and neonate

Medication	First trimester	Second and third trimesters, labor, and delivery
THYROID THERAPY Antithyroid medications: carbimazole methimazole (Tapazole) propylthiouracil	Risk of goiter and hypothyroidism; propylthiouracil is agent of choice in pregnancy.	*4, 18*
Iodides	Contraindicated in pregnancy; risk of goiter, thyroid enlargement, hypothyroidism, and mental retardation. Caution: Over-the-counter cough medications containing iodides should be avoided.	*4, 8*
TOBACCO	Intrauterine growth retardation, possible risk of spontaneous abortion, developmental delays	*3, 13*

References

1. Jones KL, Smith DW, Streissguth AP, et al. Outcome in offspring of chronic alcoholic women. *Lancet* 1:1076, 1974.

2. Clarren SR and Smith DW. The fetal alcohol syndrome. *N Engl J Med* 298:1063, 1978.

3. Beeley L. Adverse effects of drugs in the first trimester. *Clin Obstet Gynaecol* 8:261, 1981.

4. Beeley L. Adverse effects of drugs in later pregnancy. *Clin Obstet Gynaecol* 8:275, 1981.

5. Vesseym NJ. Occupational hazards of anaesthesia. *Br Med J* 281:696, 1980.

6. Perriss BW. Analgesia and anaesthesia. *Clin Obstet Gynaecol* 8:507, 1981.

7. Hall JG, Pauli RM, and Wilson KM. Maternal and fetal sequelae of anticoagulation during pregnancy. *Am J Med* 68:122, 1980.

8. Blake JP. Drugs in pregnancy: Weighing the risks. *Pat Care* 14(10):22, 1980.

9. Burrow G and Ferrio T. *Medical Complications During Pregnancy.* Philadelphia: Saunders, 1982.

10. Shepard TH. Teratogenicity of therapeutic agents. *Curr Prob Pediatr* 10(2):1, 1979.

11. Janz D. The teratogenic risk of antiepileptic drugs. *Epilepsia* 16:159, 1975.

12. Berkowitz R, Coustan D, and Mochizuki T. *Handbook for Prescribing Medications During Pregnancy.* Boston: Little, Brown, 1981.

13. Harris MC and Ericson AJ. Effect of maternal drugs on the fetus. In *Manual of Neonatal Care,* Cloherty JP and Stark AR, eds. Boston: Little, Brown, 1980.

14. Darling MR and Hawkins DF. Sex hormones in pregnancy. *Clin Obstet Gynaecol* 8:405, 1981.

15. Nora JJ and Nora AH. Birth defects and oral contraceptives. *Lancet* 1:941, 1973.

16. Sidhu RJ and Hawkins DF. Corticosteroids. *Clin Obstet Gynaecol* 8:383, 1981.

17. Friend JR. Diabetes. *Clin Obstet Gynaecol* 8:353, 1981.

18. Gurr WA. Thyroid disease. *Clin Obstet Gynaecol* 8:341, 1981.

19. Kopelman AE, McCullan FW, and Heggeness L. Limb malformations following maternal use of haloperidol. *JAMA* 231:62, 1975.

20. Mizrahi EM, Hobbs J, and Goldsmith D. Nephrogenic diabetes insipidus in transplacental lithium intoxication. *J Pediatr* 94:493, 1979.

Drugs in
Breast Milk

COMMON MEDICATIONS AFFECTING LACTATION[1]

MEDICATIONS THAT STIMULATE LACTATION

Chlorprothixene (Taractan)
Codeine
Haloperidol (Haldol)
Methyldopa
Morphine
Phenothiazines—chlorpromazine, fluphenazine, promazine (Sparine),
                thioridazine (Mellaril), and trifluoperazine (Stelazine)
Progesterone
Reserpine
Thyroid-releasing hormone
Tricyclic antidepressants

MEDICATIONS THAT INHIBIT LACTATION

Barbiturates in high doses
Bromocriptine (Parlodel)
Levodopa (Larodopa, Sinemet)
Monoamine oxidase inhibitors
Pyridoxine in high doses
Sex steroids

MEDICATIONS CONTRAINDICATED IN NURSING [2-8]

Medication	Potential effects on nursing infants
Alcohol (chronic excessive ingestion)	Hypoprothrombinemia, pseudo-Cushing syndrome, drowsiness, vomiting
Amantadine (Symmetrel)	Urinary retention, vomiting, rash
Benzodiazepines	Sedation, failure to thrive, jaundice; high doses taken regularly should be avoided.
Bromides	Sedation, rash
Chloramphenicol (Chloromycetin)	Bone marrow depression
Chlorthalidone	Possible accumulation due to long half-life; alternate medication is advisable.
Cytotoxic medications	Risk of toxicity with most agents; breast feeding is not advisable.
Dapsone	Risk of hemolytic anemia, especially in infants with G6PD deficiency
Ergotamine	Crude ergot preparations have been associated with vomiting, diarrhea, circulatory disturbance, and seizure. Risk with newer preparations—ergotamine, ergonovine, methylergonovine (Methergine) is unknown.

MEDICATIONS CONTRAINDICATED *continued*

Medication	Potential effects on nursing infants
Gold	Small quantities found in infant's serum and urine; potentially toxic.
Iodides	Hypothyroidism, goiter
Laxatives	Diarrhea with certain anthraquinones, including cascara and danthron
Lithium	Hypotonia, lethargy, cyanosis, ECG changes
Metronidazole (Flagyl)	Anorexia, vomiting, blood dyscrasias, carcinogenic in rodents
Nitrofurantoin	Risk of hemolytic anemia, especially in infants with G6PD deficiency
Radiopharmaceuticals	Contraindicated
Sulfonamides	Risk of hemolytic anemia, especially in infants with G6PD deficiency; jaundice, especially with long-acting sulfonamides

MEDICATIONS USED WITH CAUTION IN NURSING[2-11]

Medication	Potential effects on nursing infants
Aminoglycosides	Probably not absorbed; risk of fungal overgrowth and diarrhea
Antithyroid medications carbimazole methimazole (Tapazole) propylthiouracil	Concentrations at high levels may affect the infant's thyroid function. Propylthiouracil is preferred agent.
Aspirin	Chronic use of high doses may cause platelet dysfunction; safer if taken after each feeding.
Barbiturates	Drowsiness; hepatic enzyme induction may affect the metabolism of endogenous steroids.
Caffeine	Jitteriness with excessive consumption
Chloral hydrate	Sedation
Chlorpromazine	Sedation
Corticosteroids	Long-term administration of doses greater than 10 mg/day may produce adrenal suppression.
Ephedrine	Irritability and sleep disturbance (one case reported)
Indomethacin (Indocin)	Seizures (one case reported)

MEDICATIONS USED WITH CAUTION *continued*

Medication	Potential effects on nursing infants
Isoniazid	Theoretical risk of CNS- and hepatotoxicity
Meprobamate	Sedation
Nalidixic acid (NegGram)	Hemolytic anemia (one case reported of an infant whose mother was uremic)
Nicotine	Jitteriness with consumption of 20 or more cigarettes/day
Nitrofurantoin	Risk of hemolytic anemia in infants with G6PD deficiency
Oral contraceptives	Case reports of gynecomastia; possible decrease in protein, fat, and minerals in milk
Penicillin	Allergic sensitization, fungal overgrowth, diarrhea
Phenylbutazone	Theoretical risk of blood dyscrasias
Phenytoin (Dilantin)	Cyanosis and methemoglobinemia (one case reported); serious acute effects are infrequent.
Propranolol (Inderal)	Minimal risk of bradycardia and hypoglycemia
Reserpine	Nasal stuffiness

Medication	Potential effects on nursing infants
Tetracycline	Minimal risk of tooth discoloration
Theophylline	Jitteriness and sleep disturbances (infrequent reports)
Thiazides	Thrombocytopenia
Thyroid hormones	Hypothyroidism may be masked (get baseline thyroid function studies prior to breast feeding).
Tolbutamide	Theoretical risk of hypoglycemia

References

1. Dikey R. Drugs affecting lactation. *Semin Perinatol* 3:279, 1979.

2. Redetzi H. Alcohol. In *Drugs in Breast Milk*, Wilson J. New York: ADIS, 1982.

3. Anderson P. Drugs and breast feeding. *Semin Perinatol* 3:271, 1979.

4. Vorherr H. Drug excretion in breast milk. *Postgrad Med* 56:97, 1974.

5. Beeley L. Drugs and breast feeding. *Clin Obstet Gynaecol* 8:291, 1981.

6. Biller J and Yeager A, eds. *The Harriet Lane Handbook* 9th ed. Chicago: Year Book, 1981.

7. Update: Drugs in breast milk. *Med Lett* 21:21, 1979.

8. Catz CS and Giacoia GP. Drugs and breast milk. *Pediatr Clin North Am* 19:15, 1972.

9. Bauer JH, Pape B, Zajicek J, et al. Propranolol in human plasma and breast milk. *Am J Cardiol* 43:860, 1979.

10. Kampmann JP, Johansen K, Hansen JM, et al. Propylthiouracil in human milk. *Lancet* 1:736, 1980.

11. Yurchak A and Jusko W. Theophylline secretion into breast milk. *Pediatrics* 57:518, 1976.

Neonatal Pharmacology

In the past, dosing schedules were based on calculations involving the patient's age, weight, and body surface area. These calculations generally did not account for the physiologic factors that influence the elimination of medications. Among these factors are developmental changes, disease states, and aberrant physiologic mechanisms. Especially with regard to the newborn, whose metabolism changes significantly throughout the first months of life, an understanding of the effect of development on drug disposition is essential to the creation of rational dosing schedules.

Contemporary pharmacokinetics has provided a greater understanding of the factors that affect absorption, distribution, and elimination of drugs. This science, combined with a greater understanding of the newborn's physiology, has led to the development of safe and effective dosing guidelines for neonates.[1]

The purpose of this section is to review the neonate's metabolic development and how it and disease states affect drug disposition.

ABSORPTION

Oral The major determinants of drug absorption (bioavailability) are gastric acidity, gastric emptying time, and disease states.

The gastric contents at birth are neutral, due to the presence of alkaline amniotic fluid. The pH falls to 1-3 within a few hours and then returns to neutral for the first 10-15 days of life. Gastric-acid secretion increases gradually, reaching adult values at approximately two years of age. Weak acids, such as phenytoin (Dilantin), indomethacin (Indocin), and phenobarbital remain ionized in this relatively alkaline pH. Because the absorption of a drug is relatively dependent on its deionization, these compounds have decreased bioavail-

ORAL DRUG BIOAVAILABILITY IN NEONATES

Normal	Delayed	Decreased	Increased
Diazepam Digoxin Theophylline Trimethoprim- sulfamethoxazole	Acetaminophen Phenytoin Rifampin	Phenobarbital (15 days)	Ampicillin Nafcillin Penicillin

ability in the newborn. Acid-labile drugs, such as penicillin, ampicillin, and nafcillin, on the other hand, have greater bioavailability in the newborn.

The gastric emptying time is prolonged, due to irregular peristalsis, which persists for the first six to eight months.[2] The gastric emptying time is also influenced by the infant's diet. Premature formula-fed infants have a slower emptying rate than infants given breast milk.[3] Medications that ordinarily are incompletely absorbed in adults may be more extensively absorbed in the newborn due to prolonged contact with the gastric mucosa.[4]

The bioavailability of fat-soluble oral vitamin E (d-alpha-tocopherol) is decreased in premature infants. This decreased absorption may be secondary to the premature infant's impaired ability to synthesize bile acids and pancreatic enzymes.[4] Increased absorption of vitamin E comes with increasing postnatal age.

Disease states may produce adverse conditions in the gut, further decreasing drug absorption. For example, the absorption of fat-soluble vitamins is impaired in infants with steatorrhea, as is the absorption of antibiotics in infants with diarrhea.[2] Hypoxia may decrease regional blood flow to the gastrointestinal tract, with a consequent reduction in drug absorption.

The bioavailability of medications commonly administered to the newborn is summarized above.

Intramuscular The amount of drug absorbed after intramuscular injection is determined by muscle contractility, muscle mass, and regional blood flow. Differences in blood flow to various muscles and in muscular contractions may cause marked variation in the rate of drug absorption.

Intramuscular absorption in the newborn depends also on the physical properties of the drug. For example, the absorption of digoxin and the aminoglycosides is erratic, while phenobarbital is rapidly absorbed. Drug absorption changes considerably during the first two weeks, reflecting the newborn's maturational changes and adaptation to extrauterine life.[2]

Percutaneous Absorption of topically applied medications is enhanced due to the newborn's thin stratum corneum. Because of the risks of neurotoxicity following the topical administration of hexachlorophene and of systemic effects after the excessive use of corticosteroids, topical medications must be used with caution.

DISTRIBUTION

Distribution is the process by which the drug separates from circulating blood and enters into the various body compartments.[5] Drug distribution influences the extent of pharmacologic activity. The factors that determine distribution include body water content, fat content, protein binding, and regional blood flow.

The total body water content is greater in newborns than in adults and older children. The ratio of extracellular to intracellular fluid volume is also greater. Accordingly, water-soluble drugs have a larger volume of distribution in newborns and may have to be given in higher doses to produce a therapeutic response. Fat content, on the other hand, is lower in newborns, and so lipid-soluble drugs have a smaller volume of distribution. The sizes of these body compartments continuously change throughout the neonatal period. Therefore, changes in drug distribution have to be expected.

The quantity of protein and the ability of protein to bind drugs are low in the newborn. In addition, drugs must compete for binding sites with compounds such as bilirubin, free fatty acids, and hormones. This may result in the displacement of bilirubin or increased concentrations of free drug. Elevated bilirubin increases the risk of kernicterus, while higher quantities of free drug produce enhanced pharmacologic activity.

Decreased protein binding of phenytoin results in free drug levels higher in infants than in adults[6]; consequently, serum concentrations that are therapeutic in adults may produce toxicity in the newborn.

The plasma protein binding of drugs doesn't reach adult values until one year of age. Therefore, alterations in drug distribution occur throughout infancy.

METABOLISM

The infant is born with low concentrations of the hepatic microsomal enzymes necessary to metabolize many drugs. Therefore, medications metabolized by these enzymes have a prolonged duration of action in the newborn. Dose adjustments must be made to prevent drug accumulation and toxicity.

Decreased glucuronic activity is due to low concentrations of the hepatic enzymes glucuronyl transferase and uridine diphosphate glucuronic dehydrogenase. Drugs excreted after conjugation with glucuronic acid include chloramphenicol, indomethacin, and salicylates.[7,8,9] The half-life of these agents is prolonged in the newborn. These drugs should be administered less frequently and in lower doses.

Sulfate conjugation processes are well-developed at birth. Acetaminophen, a drug conjugated by glucuronic activity in adults, is eliminated as a sulfate metabolite in infants.[10] The ability of the newborn to use an alternative pathway results in a half-life for this drug similar to that observed in adults.

Newborns have a limited ability to metabolize drugs such as phenobarbital, phenytoin, and diazepam (Valium), and so the rate of elimination of these drugs is prolonged. Accumulation of diazepam and its active metabolites may cause undesirable effects in infants of mothers receiving large doses during labor.[2]

Exposure to enzyme inducers, in utero or shortly after birth, enhances the activity of hepatic microsomal enzymes. Phenobarbital, phenytoin, and carbamazepine (Tegretol) are potent enzyme-inducing agents. Serum levels of phenobarbital and phenytoin must be monitored to avoid seizure activity, which may result from subtherapeutic levels.

Postnatal age, pathology, and previous exposure to enzyme inducers influence the rate of hepatic maturation. The initial phase of low metabolic activity is followed by an increase in enzyme activity that surpasses the metabolic capacity of adults. Adult rates of metabolism occur at about two or three years of age. Thus the infant goes from being at risk for overdose to being at risk for inadequate medication. Monitoring drug levels in serum is necessary for designing a dosing regimen that is safe and effective for the individual patient.

RENAL ELIMINATION

One or more of three mechanisms influence the renal excretion of drugs: glomerular filtration, tubular secretion, and tubular reabsorption.[4] Glomerular filtration develops most rapidly in the newborn, followed by tubular secretion, and more slowly by tubular reabsorption. The factors that affect the rate of renal maturation have not been clearly defined. Renal development is correlated with postnatal age, but further studies are needed to clarify its relationship to gestational age and previous drug exposure. Disease states that modify renal blood flow will delay maturation and possibly further diminish renal function.

The glomerular filtration rate in a newborn is 30 percent of that measured in adults.[10] Investigators, using inulin and aminohippuric acid clearance, have documented a twofold increase in the glomerular filtration rate by two weeks of age.[11] Adult values are not achieved until about one year of age.[4] Medications eliminated by glomerular filtration have increased rates of clearance in the first few weeks of life. Based on this fact, doses of penicillin, ampicillin, and aminoglycosides should be increased after the first week of life.

CONCLUSION

Research in the disciplines of developmental physiology and pharmacokinetics has resulted in the development of dosing recommendations for the neonate. A summary of the information is presented in the following sections.

Although dosing guidelines are available, because of the unpredictable development of organs responsible for drug disposition, it's necessary to monitor serum concentrations of medications with narrow therapeutic indices. Medications that should be monitored include the aminoglycosides, chloramphenicol, vancomycin (Vancocin), caffeine, theophylline, phenobarbital, and phenytoin. The therapeutic ranges for these medications have been included in this book.

References

1. Morselli PL, Franco-Morselli R, and Bossi L. Clinical pharmacokinetics in newborns and infants. *Clin Pharmacokinet* 5:485, 1980.

2. Shirkey HC. Pediatric clinical pharmacology and therapeutics. In *Drug Treatment Principles and Practice of Clinical Pharmacology and Therapeutics,* Avery GS, ed. New York: ADIS, 1980.

3. Cavell B. Gastric emptying time in preterm infants. *Acta Paediatr Scand* 68:723, 1979.

4. Hilligoss DM. Neonatal pharmacokinetics. In *Applied Pharmacokinetics,* Evans W, Schentag J, and Jusko W, eds. San Francisco: Applied Therapeutics, 1980.

5. Lesko LJ. Pharmacokinetics of drugs in the neonate. *Apothecary* 90:30, 1978.

6. Loughnan PM, Greenwald A, Purton WW, et al. Pharmacokinetic observations of phenytoin disposition in the newborn and young infant. *Arch Dis Child* 52:302, 1977.

7. Lietman PS. Chloramphenicol and the neonate: 1979. *Clin Pharmacol* 6:151, 1979.

8. Yaffe SJ, Friedman WF, Rogers D, et al. The disposition of indomethacin in preterm babies. *J Pediatr* 97:1001, 1980.

9. Morselli PL. Clinical pharmacokinetics in neonates. *Clin Pharmacokinet* 1:81, 1976.

10. Miller RP, Roberts RJ, and Fischer LJ. Acetaminophen elimination kinetics in neonates, children, and adults. *Clin Pharmacol Ther* 19:284, 1976.

11. Guignard JP, Torrado A, DeCunha O, et al. Glomerular filtration rate in the first three weeks of life. *J Pediatr* 87:268, 1975.

Antimicrobial Drug Therapy

ANTIMICROBIAL THERAPY

Drug	Dosage (parenteral, except as noted)	
Amikacin (Amikin)	**0-7 days**	**>7 days** [1]
	7.5 mg/kg every 12 hours	7.5 mg/kg every 12 hours (<2 kg)
		7.5 mg/kg every 8 hours (>2 kg)
Amphotericin B (Fungizone)	All infants: 0.25 mg-1.0 mg/kg/day [2,4,5] (after test dose of 0.1 mg/kg) via slow IV drip over 2-6 hours; concentration of infusate should not exceed 0.1 mg/ml	
Ampicillin	**0-7 days**	**>7 days** [1]
	25 mg/kg every 12 hours	25 mg/kg every 8 hours
	50 mg/kg every 12 hours (in meningitis)	50 mg/kg every 6 hours (in meningitis)
Carbenicillin (Geopen)	**0-7 days**	**>7 days** [1,3]
	100 mg/kg every 12 hours	100 mg/kg every 8 hours (<2 kg)
		100 mg/kg every 6 hours (>2 kg)

Therapeutic range	Side effects	Comment
Trough: *2* <10 mcg/ml Peak: 15-25 mcg/ml <30 mcg/ml (>2 kg)	Nephrotoxicity,** ototoxicity,** neuromuscular blockade after anesthesia and concomitant use with muscle relaxants	Renal toxicity and ototoxicity associated with elevated peak and trough levels. Reduce dosage in patients with renal dysfunction.
N/A	Phlebitis, fever, nephrotoxicity, *6* anemia, hypokalemia	
N/A	Rash, gastrointestinal disturbances, *3* twitching and seizures**	
N/A	Hypernatremia, hypokalemia, *4* inhibition of platelet aggregation	

**Toxic manifestations.

Drug	Dosage (parenteral, except as noted)	
Cefazolin* (Ancef, Kefzol)		2,3
	0-7 days	**>7 days**
	25 mg/kg every 12 hours	25 mg/kg every 8 hours
Cefotaxime* (Claforan)	Premature infants:	7
	0-7 days	**>7 days**
	25 mg/kg every 12 hours	25 mg/kg every 8 hours
	Full-term infants:	
	25 mg/kg every 8 hours	25 mg/kg every 6 hours
Cephalothin* (Keflin)	All infants: 25 mg/kg every 6 hours	4
Chloramphenicol sodium succinate		1
	0-14 days	**15-30 days**
	25 mg/kg every 24 hours	25 mg/kg every 24 hours (<2 kg)
		25 mg/kg every 12 hours (>2 kg and infants <2 kg with meningitis)
Erythromycin*	All infants: 5 mg/kg IV, PO, every 6 hours	4

*Limited data concerning use in newborns.

34

Therapeutic range	Side effects		Comment
N/A	See cefotaxime		
N/A	Leukopenia, neutropenia, transient elevation of SGOT and BUN		These side effects have been noted in adults.
N/A	See cefotaxime		
10-25 mcg/ml; time of sample: at least 6 hours after the dose	Dose-related bone marrow suppression,** idiosyncratic aplastic anemia, gray baby syndrome**	8	Tests for monitoring bone marrow suppression: reticulocyte count, serum iron, TIBC, CBC
N/A	GI disturbances, cholestasia (rare and reported only in use of estolate salt); parenteral administration may be painful.	3	

**Toxic manifestations.

Drug	Dosage (parenteral, except as noted)	
Flucytosine (Ancobon)	All infants: 100-150 mg/kg/day PO in 4 divided doses	5
Gentamicin	**0-7 days** **>7 days** 2.5 mg/kg 2.5 mg/kg every 12 hours every 8 hours 2.5 mg/kg every 6 hours PO in necrotizing enterocolitis	3,9
Isoniazid*	All infants: 10 mg/kg/day PO, prophylaxis 15-30 mg/kg/day, therapy	2,4

*Limited data concerning use in newborns.

Therapeutic range	Side effects		Comment
N/A	Thrombocytopenia, leukopenia, aplastic anemia, elevated liver enzyme tests	6	Side effects are uncommon. Organisms become resistant when this drug is used alone.
Trough: <2 mcg/ml Peak: 4-8 mcg/ml Time of samples— trough: prior to the next dose; peak: IV, ½ hour after the infusion; IM, 1 hour after the dose 2	Nephrotoxicity,** ototoxicity,** neuromuscular blockade after anesthesia and concomitant administration of muscle relaxants	3	Renal 9 toxicity and ototoxicity associated with elevated peak and trough levels. De-crease dose in patients with renal dysfunc-tion. There is controversy over use of the oral drug in necrotizing enterocolitis.
N/A	Hepatotoxicity, B_6 depletion	4	

**Toxic manifestations.

Drug	Dosage (parenteral, except as noted)	
Kanamycin		*1, 10*
	0-7 days	**>7 days**
	7.5 mg/kg every 12 hours (<2 kg)	10 mg/kg every 12 hours (<2 kg)
	10 mg/kg every 12 hours (>2 kg)	10 mg/kg every 8 hours (>2 kg)
	15 mg/kg/day PO in 3 divided doses in necrotizing enterocolitis	
Methicillin (Staphcillin)		*1,2*
	0-14 days	**15-30 days**
	25 mg/kg every 12 hours (<2 kg)	25-50 mg/kg every 8 hours (<2 kg)
	25 mg/kg every 8 hours (>2 kg)	25-50 mg/kg every 6 hours (>2 kg)
Metronidazole* (Flagyl)	Loading dose: 15 mg/kg *11*	
	Maintenance dose	
	0-7 days	**>7 days**
	7.5 mg/kg every 12 hours	7.5 mg/kg every 12 hours

*Limited data concerning use in newborns.

Therapeutic range	Side effects		Comment
Trough: 2 2-4 mcg/ml Peak: 15-25 mcg/ml Time of samples: See gentamicin	See gentamicin	2	See gentamicin
N/A	Nephrotoxicity,** seizures	3	Nephrotoxicity is rare in the newborn.
N/A	Seizures,** dark urine, GI disturbances, reversible neutropenia, thrombophlebitis		These side effects have been noted in adults.

**Toxic manifestations.

Drug	Dosage (parenteral, except as noted)		

Mezlocillin* (Mezlin) — 12

0-7 days	>7 days
75 mg/kg every 12 hours	75 mg/kg every 8 hours (<2 kg)
	75 mg/kg every 6 hours (>2 kg)

Moxalactam — 13

0-6 days	7-28 days	>28 days
50 mg/kg every 12 hours	50 mg/kg every 8 hours	50 mg/kg every 4 hours

In meningitis, administer a loading dose of 100 mg/kg.

Nafcillin* (Nafcil, Unipen) — 2

0-7 days	>7 days
50-100 mg/kg/day in 2 divided doses	100-200 mg/kg/day in 3 or 4 divided doses

Nystatin — 3

All infants: 100,000-200,000 units PO every 6 hours

*Limited data concerning use in newborns.

Therapeutic range	Side effects		Comment
N/A	Hypokalemia, transient elevation of SGOT, SGPT, alkaline phosphatase, bilirubin	12	
N/A	Prolonged bleeding time, neutropenia, eosinophilia, transient elevations in renal or liver function tests	14	
N/A	Transient neutropenia		
N/A	Vomiting, diarrhea		

ANTIMICROBIAL THERAPY *continued*

Drug	Dosage (parenteral, except as noted)	
Oxacillin	**0-7 days** 50-100 mg/kg/day in 2 divided doses	**>7 days** 100-200 mg/kg/day in 3 or 4 divided doses
Penicillin G	[1,2] **0-7 days** 25,000 units/kg every 12 hours 50,000-75,000 units/kg every 12 hours (meningitis)	**>7 days** 25,000 units/kg every 8 hours 50,000-75,000 units/kg every 6 hours (meningitis)
Penicillin G procaine	All infants: 50,000 units/kg/day [1]	
Pyrimethamine (Daraprim)	All infants: 2 mg/kg/day PO in 2 divided [16] doses for 72 hours; 1 mg/kg/day PO in 2 divided doses for 28 days	

Therapeutic range	Side effects		Comment
N/A	Transient neutropenia, elevation of alkaline phosphatase and SGOT	14	
N/A	Neutropenia, seizures**	16	Increased risk of seizures at doses >250,000 units/kg/day
N/A	See penicillin G		
N/A	Folic acid deficiency, bone marrow suppression	4, 16	Administer 16 folinic acid, 1 mg/kg/day; Monitor reticulocyte count, CBC, platelet count.

**Toxic manifestations.

Drug	Dosage (parenteral, except as noted)	
Rifampin (Rifadin)	All infants: 10-20 mg/kg/day PO	*3,17*
Sulfadiazine (Suladyne)	All infants: 100-150 mg/kg/day PO in 4 divided doses	*16*

Ticarcillin* (Ticar)   *18*

Loading dose: 100 mg/kg

Maintenance dose

0-7 days	7-14 days	>14 days (>2 kg)
75 mg/kg every 8 hours (<2 kg)	75 mg/kg every 4-6 hours	100 mg/kg every 4 hours
75 mg/kg every 6 hours (>2 kg)		

*Limited data concerning use in newborns.

Therapeutic range	Side effects	Comment
N/A	Vomiting, diarrhea, thrombocytopenia, leukopenia, anemia, hepatotoxicity, red-orange discoloration of body fluids *3*	Organisms rapidly become resistant when this drug is used alone.
N/A	Crystalluria, hematuria, hyperbilirubinemia, bone marrow suppression *16*	
N/A	Hypernatremia, hypokalemia, decreased platelet aggregation *16*	

Drug	Dosage (parenteral, except as noted)	
Tobramycin (Nebcin)	**0-7 days**	2,18,19 **>7 days**
	2.5 mg/kg every 24 hours (<1.5 kg)	2.5 mg/kg every 12 hours (<2 kg)
	2.5 mg/kg every 18 hours (1.5-2.0 kg)	2.5 mg/kg every 8 hours (>2 kg)
	2.5 mg/kg every 12 hours (>2 kg)	
Vancomycin (Vancocin)	**0-7 days**	4,20 **>7 days**
	15 mg/kg every 12 hours	15 mg/kg every 8 hours
Vidarabine (Vira-A)	All infants: 15 mg/kg/day IV over 12 hours; 21,22 concentration of solution ≤0.7 mg/ml	

Therapeutic range	Side effects	Comment
Trough: *2* <2 mcg/ml Peak: 4-8 mcg/ml Time of samples: See gentamicin	Nephrotoxicity,** ototoxicity,** neuromuscular blockade after anesthesia and concomitant administration of muscle relaxants	Renal toxicity and ototoxicity associated with elevated peak and trough levels. Decrease dose in patients with renal dysfunction.
Trough: *2,16* 5-10 mcg/ml Peak: 25-30 mcg/ml	Ototoxicity,** nephrotoxicity,** *20* phlebitis	Ototoxicity occurs with serum levels >30 mcg/ml
N/A	Bone marrow megaloblastosis, *22* weight loss, leukopenia, neutropenia, thrombocytopenia	These side effects have been noted in adults.

**Toxic manifestations.

References

1. McCracken GH, Nelson JD, and Oliver T, eds. *Antimicrobial Therapy for Newborns.* New York: Grune & Stratton, 1977.

2. Blumer JL and Blumenfeld TA. Therapeutic agents. In *Behrman's Neonatal-Perinatal Medicine,* 3rd ed, Fanaroff AA and Martin RJ, eds. St. Louis: Mosby, 1983.

3. Eichenwald HR and McCracken GH. Antimicrobial therapy in infants and children. *J Pediatr* 93:337, 1978.

4. Avery GB, ed. *Neonatology.* Philadelphia: Lippincott, 1981.

5. Lillen L, Ramamurth YR, and Pildes R. *Candida albicans* meningitis in a premature neonate successfully treated with 5-fluorocytosine and amphotericin B: A case report and review of the literature. *Pediatrics* 61:57, 1978.

6. Chesney PJ, Teets KC, Mulvihill JJ, et al. Successful treatment of *Candida* meningitis with amphotericin B and 5-fluorocytosine in combination. *J Pediatr* 89:1017, 1976.

7. Kafetzis DA, Brater DC, Kapiki AN, et al. Treatment of severe neonatal infections with cefotaxime: Efficacy and pharmacokinetics. *J Pediatr* 100:483, 1982.

8. Dajani A and Kauffman R. The renaissance of chloramphenicol. *Pediatr Clin North Am* 28:195, 1981.

9. Grylack L and Scanlon J. Oral gentamicin therapy in the prevention of necrotizing enterocolitis. *Am J Dis Child* 32:1192, 1981.

10. Egan EA, Mantilla G, Nelson RM, et al. A prospective controlled trial of oral kanamycin in the prevention of neonatal necrotizing enterocolitis. *J Pediatr* 89:467, 1976.

11. Jager-Roman E, Doyle PE, Baird-Lambert J, et al. Pharmacokinetics and tissue distribution of metronidazole in the newborn infant. *J Pediatr* 100:651, 1982.

12. Nelson J and McCracken GH. Mezlocillin and related antibiotics. *Pediatr Infect Dis* 1:42, 1982.

13. Schaad UB, McCracken GH, Threlkeld N, et al. Clinical evaluation of a new broad-spectrum oxa-beta-lactam antibiotic, moxalactam, in neonates and infants. *J Pediatr* 98:129, 1981.

14. Levy RL and Saunders RL. Citrobacter meningitis in cerebral abscess in early infancy: Cure by moxalactam. *Neurology* 31:1575, 1981.

15. Baker C. Group B streptococcus infections in neonates. *Pediatr Rev* 1:5, 1979.

16. Mandel G, Douglas R, and Bennett J, eds. *Principles and Practice of Infectious Diseases*. New York: Wiley, 1980.

17. Acocella G. Clinical pharmacokinetics of rifampin. *Clin Pharmacokinet* 3:108, 1978.

18. Nelson JD, Shelton S, and Kusmiesz H. Clinical pharmacology of ticarcillin in the newborn infant: Relation to age, gestational age, and weight. *J Pediatr* 87:474, 1975.

19. Arbeter AM, Sacoar CL, Eisner S, et al. Tobramycin sulfate elimination in premature infants. *J Pediatr* 103:131, 1983.

20. Schaad UB, McCracken GH, and Nelson JD. Clinical pharmacology and efficacy of vancomycin in pediatric patients. *J Pediatr* 96:119, 1980.

21. Whitley R, Nahmias AJ, Soong SJ, et al. Vidarabine therapy for neonatal herpes simplex virus infection. *Pediatrics* 66:495, 1980.

22. Liu C. Antiviral drugs. *Med Clin North Am* 66:235, 1982.

Cardiovascular Drug Therapy

Medication	Indication	Dosage/route	
Acetazolamide	Hypertension, edema	5 mg/kg/day PO	1,2
Alprostadil	Ductus arteriosus-dependent congenital heart disease	0.05-0.1 mcg/kg/min IV Maximum dose: 0.4 mcg/kg/min	3,4

Therapeutic range	Side effects			Comment
N/A	Hypokalemia, metabolic acidosis		2	
N/A	**Reported side effect**	**Incidence**	5 **Risk factors**	Decrease dose to the lowest infusion rate needed to maintain a therapeutic response.

	Cardiovascular*
	  cutaneous
	  vasodilation
	  edema
	  arrhythmias
	  hypotension
		18%	Intra-arterial administration, infants <2 kg, duration of therapy >48 hours	

	Central nervous system
	  seizures
	  fever*
		16%	Pre-infusion pH <7.15, duration of therapy >48 hours	

	Respiratory*
	  depression
	  apnea
		12%	Infants <2 kg, cyanosis	

	Metabolic
	  hypoglycemia
	  hypocalcemia
		2%		

	Infection	2%	Infants <2 kg	
	GI disturbances	2%		

	Hematologic**
	  DIC
	  thrombo-
	    cytopenia
	  hemorrhage
		2%		

	Renal failure**	2%		

*Side effect secondary to drug therapy.
**Questionable relation to drug therapy.

Medication	Indication	Dosage/route
Atropine	Bradycardia, AV block	0.01-0.03 mg/kg IV *6,7*
Calcium gluconate	Low cardiac output	100 mg/kg IV over *1,7* 5-10 min
Captopril (Capoten)	Hypertension	0.1-0.4 mg/kg PO *8* 1-4 times a day
Chlorothiazide	Hypertension	10-20 mg/kg/day *1,2* PO in divided doses every 12 hours
Diazoxide (Hyperstat)	Hypertensive crisis	2-5 mg/kg rapid *9,10* IV infusion (over 30 sec) May repeat in 4-8 hours if needed. *Note: Administer 2* *mg/kg to patients* *with hypoalbuminemia* *or contracted* *intravascular space*

Therapeutic range	Side effects	Comment
N/A	Hyperthermia, urinary retention, tachycardia *1*	
N/A	Bradycardia, arrhythmias *7*	Monitor ECG.
N/A	Proteinuria, hyperkalemia, hypotension, agranulocytosis (rare) *8*	These side effects have been noted in adults; limited data concerning use in newborns.
N/A	Electrolyte abnormalities: hypokalemia, hyponatremia, hypercalcemia *2* Hyperglycemia, hyperuricemia (rare), metabolic alkalosis, interstitial nephritis (uncommon)	
N/A	Sodium and water retention, hypotension, hyperglycemia, increased levels of free fatty acids *9,10*	Not indicated for maintenance therapy; contraindicated in patients with aortic coarctation

Medication	Indication	Dosage/route
Digoxin	Congestive heart failure, supraventricular arrhythmias	*11,12,13,14* **Total digitalizing dose** Premature: 0.02 mg/kg IV Full-term: 0.02-0.04 mg/kg IV, 0.03-0.05 mg/kg PO Infant >1 month: 0.04-0.05 mg/kg PO **Maintenance dose** Premature: 0.005-0.01 mg/kg/day PO Full-term: 0.01 mg/kg/day PO Infants >1 month: 0.015-0.025 mg/kg/day PO *Note: IV dose is ¾ of the oral dose.*

Therapeutic range	Side effects		Comment
		15, 16, 17	15, 16
0.8-2 ng/ml. Time of sample, trough level: prior to the next dose. *Note: All digoxin levels must be drawn at least 8 hours after the last dose.*	**Toxicities** Vomiting Poor feeding Bradycardia AV block Arrhythmias (PVCs)	**Risk factors** Hypokalemia Hypomagnesemia Hypercalcemia Acidosis Renal disease Hypothyroidism Interactions with indomethacin, diuretics, quinidine, verapamil, caffeine	**Management of toxicity:** 1. Discontinue digoxin. 2. Draw a serum digoxin level. 3. Correct electrolyte abnormalities. 4. In acute oral overdoses, administer cholestyramine(Questran) or kaolin (Kaolin-Pectin). 5. Specific binding antibodies 6. Arrhythmias, AV block: atropine, propranolol; ventricular: phenytoin, lidocaine, procainamide 7. Hemoperfusion

Medication	Indication	Dosage/route
Dobutamine (Dobutrex)	Cardiovascular shock	2.5-7.5 mcg/kg/min IV [18]
Dopamine	Hypotension, shock	2-20 mcg/kg/min IV [20]

Dopamine dosage/effect:

Dosage	Effect
2-5 mcg/kg/min	↑ Renal blood flow
5-15 mcg/kg/min	↑ Renal blood flow ↑ Heart rate ↑ Cardiac contractility
>20 mcg/kg/min	↓ Renal blood flow ↑ Heart rate ↑ Cardiac contractility Vasoconstriction

Medication	Indication	Dosage/route
Epinephrine	Asystole, bradycardia	0.1 ml/kg of a 1:10,000 solution IV,IC; may repeat in 5 min [6]

Therapeutic range	Side effects	Comment
N/A	Hypotension, hypertension, [18,19] arrhythmias (sinus tachycardia and ventricular tachycardia), increased pulmonary wedge pressure with pulmonary edema *Note: side effects most common at doses >7.5 mcg/kg/min.*	Correct [18,19] hypovolemia, electrolytes, and acid-base balance prior to therapy.
N/A	Sinus tachycardia, ventricular [1,19] irritability, peripheral ischemia (high doses), pulmonary hypertension	Correct hypovolemia, electrolytes, and acid-base balance prior to therapy.
N/A	Hypertension, ventricular fibrillation [7]	

Medication	Indication	Dosage/route
Furosemide	Symptomatic patent ductus arteriosus, congestive heart failure, edema, hypercalcemia, bronchopulmonary dysplasia, hyaline membrane disease	1-2 mg/kg IV; [21,22,23] may repeat in 8-24 hours as needed. *Note: Bioavailability with oral administration <20%*
Hydralazine	Hypertension	1-9 mg/kg/day [24] IV, PO in 4 divided doses
Indomethacin (Indocin)	Closure of the patent ductus arteriosus	0.1-0.3 mg/kg PO; [25] may repeat if needed in 12-24 hours × 3 doses
	Note: Studies report results of the IV formulation indomethacin, which is under investigation. The FDA has approved indomethacin only for oral administration.	
Isoproterenol	Heart block, bradycardia, cardiogenic shock	Initial IV infusion: [1,30] 0.05-0.1 mcg/kg/min; titrate dose to desired response

Therapeutic range	Side effects	Comment
N/A	Electrolyte abnormalities [1,2] (hyponatremia and hypokalemia), dehydration, metabolic alkalosis, hyperglycemia, displacement of bilirubin, interstitial nephritis (rare), ototoxicity (with serum levels >25 mcg/ml), nephrocalcinosis, hepatic necrosis (rare)	Perinatal asphyxia may decrease response to furosemide. Use of furosemide for hyaline membrane disease is controversial.
N/A	Tachycardia, hypotension, sodium [1,24] and water retention, diarrhea, vomiting, hematologic abnormalities (rare)	
A level [26] >250 mg/ml at 24 hours has been associated with increased response.	Transient oliguria, increased [27,28,29] serum creatinine, inhibition of platelet aggregation, thrombocytopenia, transient decrease of serum sodium, transient increase of serum potassium, transient ileus	Contra-indications: overt bleeding, coagulation abnormality, serum creatinine >1.6 mg/dl, necrotizing enterocolitis
N/A	Increased heart rate, arrhythmias, [7] decreased cardiac output if heart rate >180-200 beats/min, hypotension	

Medication	Indication	Dosage/route
Lidocaine	Ventricular arrhythmias	IV bolus: 1-2 mg/kg [31] over 5 min; may repeat dose to a maximum cumulative dose of 5 mg/kg IV infusion: 10-25 mcg/kg/min
Methyldopa	Hypertension	5-50 mg/kg/day IV, [24] PO in 3 divided doses
Nitroprusside (Nipride, Nitropress)	Hypertension, heart failure	0.5-8 mcg/kg/min IV [9]
Procainamide	Used rarely to treat specific rhythm disturbances	Inital IV [31,32,33] dose: 3-6 mg/kg over 5 min to 500 mg Maintenance IV dose: 20-80 mcg/kg/min 15-50 mg/kg/day PO divided into 4-6 doses

Therapeutic range	Side effects	Comment
N/A	Hypotension, lethargy,* seizures,* respiratory arrest,* coma* *31*	
N/A	Lethargy, hypotension, sodium and water retention, positive direct Coombs' test (without hemolysis), hemolytic anemia, hepatotoxicity (rare)—abnormal liver function tests, cholestasis, jaundice, chronic hepatitis *1,9,24*	
9 Thiocyanate level <10 mg/dl	Hypotension, tachyphylaxis, thiocyanate toxicity*—hypoplasia, muscle spasm, weakness, bone marrow suppression (rare), hypothyroidism—cyanide toxicity* *1,9*	Keep bottle covered to avoid photodegradation.
3-10 31 mcg/ml	Hypotension, arrhythmias (ventricular tachycardia and ventricular fibrillation), nausea, vomiting, seizures, thrombocytopenia, agranulocytosis *31,33*	Limited data concerning use in the newborn

*Toxic manifestations.

Medication	Indication	Dosage/route
Propranolol (Inderal)	Hypertension, supraventricular tachycardia	Hypertension: [19,24,32] 0.5-2 mg/kg/day PO divided into 3 or 4 doses Supraventricular tachycardia: 0.05-0.15 mg/kg Administer half the calculated dose IV at a rate <1 mg/min; repeat in 2 minutes if needed.
Quinidine	Used rarely to treat [1] specific rhythm disturbances	15-40 mg/kg/day PO [31] in 4 divided doses
Sodium bicarbonate	Metabolic acidosis *Note: mEq of bicarbonate = body weight (kg) $\times$ base deficit $\times$ 0.3*	1-2 mEq/kg IV [1] Subsequent doses are calculated on base deficit.

Therapeutic range	Side effects	Comment
N/A	Bradycardia, asystole, [1,33,34] bronchospasm, hypoglycemia, hypotension, congestive heart failure	Monitor ECG during administration. Treat bradycardia with atropine.
2.5-6.0 [31] mcg/ml	Hypotension, depressed atrial [31] activity,* arrhythmias* (ventricular tachycardia, ventricular flutter, and ventricular fibrillation), asystole,* vomiting, tremor, seizures, thrombocytopenia, anemia	Discontinue if QRS interval >0.1 sec. Limited data concerning use in newborns
N/A	Transient hyperosmolarity, alkalosis [1]	Contraindicated in respiratory acidosis

*Toxic manifestations.

Medication	Indication	Dosage/route
Spironolactone	Edema secondary to congestive heart failure or liver disease	0.5-1.0 mg/kg PO [1] every 8 hours
Verapamil (Calan, Isoptin)	Supraventricular tachycardia	0.15-0.4 mg/kg IV; [35] no data on maintenance dose

Therapeutic range	Side effects		Comment
N/A	Hyperkalemia	*1*	
N/A	Bradycardia, AV block, asystole	*35*	*35,36* Contraindications: hypocalcemia, concomitant administration of beta-blockers

CARDIAC RESUSCITATION DRUGS

Drug	Indication	Dosage IV
Atropine	Bradycardia	0.01-0.03 mg/kg; may repeat in 20 minutes
Calcium gluconate	Low cardiac output	100 mg/kg over 5-10 min
Dopamine	Hypotension	5 mcg/kg/min; increase to achieve desired response
Epinephrine	Bradycardia, asystole	0.1 ml/kg of a 1:10,000 solution; may repeat in 5-10 min
Isoproterenol	Low cardiac output, bradycardia	0.1 mcg/kg/min; titrate infusion rate to achieve desired response
Lidocaine	Ventricular arrhythmias	Bolus: 1 mg/kg over 5 min Infusion: 10-50 mcg/kg/min
Naloxone (Narcan)	Reversal of narcotic depression	0.01 mg/kg; may repeat every 10-15 min as needed
Sodium bicarbonate	Metabolic acidosis	1-2 mEq/kg; adjust according to pH

References

1. Avery B, ed. *Neonatology.* Philadelphia: Lippincott, 1981.

2. Bailie MD, Linshaw MA, and Stygles VG. Diuretic pharmacology in infants and children. *Pediatr Clin North Am* 28:217, 1981.

3. Prostin VR Pediatric. Kalamazoo, Mich: Upjohn, 1981.

4. Freed MD, Heymann MA, Lewis AB, et al. Prostaglandin E_1 in infants with ductus arteriosus-dependent congenital heart disease. *Circulation* 64:899, 1981.

5. Lewis AB, Freed MD, Heymann MA, et al. Side effects of therapy with prostaglandin E_1 in infants with critical congenital heart disease. *Circulation* 64:893, 1981.

6. Standards and guidelines for cardiopulmonary resuscitation (CPR) and emergency cardiac care, Part V: Advanced cardiac life support for neonates. *JAMA* 244:495, 1980.

7. Gregory G. Resuscitation of the newborn. *Anesthesiology* 43:225, 1975.

8. Bifano E, Post EM, Springer J, et al. Treatment of neonatal hypertension with captopril. *J Pediatr* 100:143, 1982.

9. Pruitt A. Pharmacologic approach to the management of childhood hypertension. *Pediatr Clin North Am* 28:135, 1981.

10. Balfe JW and Rance CP. Recognition and management of hypertensive crises in childhood. *Pediatr Clin North Am* 25:159, 1978.

11. Pinsky WW, Jacobsen JR, Gillette PC, et al. Dosage of digoxin in premature infants. *J Pediatr* 94:639, 1979.

12. Halkin H, Radomsky M, Blieden L, et al. Steady-state serum digoxin concentration in relation to digitalis toxicity in neonates and infants. *Pediatrics* 61:184, 1978.

13. Nyberg L and Wettrell G. Pharmacokinetics and dosage of digoxin in neonates and infants. *Eur J Clin Pharmacol* 18:69, 1980.

14. Morselli PL, Morselli RF, and Bosei L. Clinical pharmacokinetics in newborns and infants. *Clin Pharmacokinet* 5:485, 1980.

15. Brshahan J and Vlietstra D. Digitalis glycosides. *Mayo Clin Proc* 54:675, 1979.

16. Soyka LF. Pediatric clinical pharmacology of digoxin. *Pediatr Clin North Am* 28:203, 1981.

17. Schimmel MS, Inwood RJ, Eidelman AL, et al. Toxic digitalis levels associated with indomethacin therapy in a neonate. *Clin Pediatr* 19:768, 1980.

18. Petkin RM, Levin DL, Webb R, et al. Dobutamine: A hemodynamic evaluation of children in shock. *J Pediatr* 100:977, 1982.

19. Latts JR and Goldberg LJ. Dopamine in the management of shock. *Drug Ther* 4:25, 1979.

20. Driscoll DJ, Gillette PC, and McNamara DG. The use of dopamine in children. *J Pediatr* 92:309, 1978.

21. Peterson RG, Simmons MA, Rumack BH, et al. Pharmacology of furosemide in the premature newborn infant. *J Pediatr* 97:139, 1980.

22. Ross BS, Pollack A, and Oh W. The pharmacologic effects of furosemide therapy in the low-birth-weight infant. *J Pediatr* 97:139, 1980.

23. Aranda JV, Turmen T, and Sasyniuk BI. Pharmacokinetics of diuretics and methylxanthines in the neonate. *Eur J Clin Pharmacol* 18:55, 1980.

24. Adelman R. Neonatal hypertension. *Pediatr Clin North Am* 25:99, 1978.

25. Clyman RI and Heymann HA. Pharmacology of the ductus arteriosus. *Pediatr Clin North Am* 28:77, 1981.

26. Brash AR, Hickey DE, Graham TP, et al. Pharmacokinetics of indomethacin in the neonate. *N Engl J Med* 305:67, 1981.

27. Vert P, Bianchetti G, Marchal F, et al. Effectiveness and pharmacokinetics of indomethacin in premature newborns with patent ductus arteriosus. *Eur J Clin Pharmacol* 18:83, 1980.

28. Yeh TF, Luken JA, Thalji A, et al. Intravenous indomethacin therapy in premature infants with persistent ductus arteriosus: A double-blind controlled study. *J Pediatr* 98:137, 1981.

29. Gersony WM, Peckham GJ, and Ellison RC. Effects of indomethacin in premature infants with patent ductus arteriosus: Results of a national collaborative study. *J Pediatr* 102:895, 1983.

30. Zenk KE and Amlie R. Neonatal emergency transport drug box. *Drug Intel Clin Pharm* 16:122, 1982.

31. Gelband H and Rosen H. Pharmacologic basis for the treatment of cardiac arrhythmias. *Pediatrics* 55:59, 1975.

32. Lees MH and Sunderland CO. The cardiovascular system. In *Behrman's Neonatal-Perinatal Medicine,* 3rd ed, Fanaroff AA and Martin RJ, eds. St. Louis: Mosby, 1983.

33. Olley P. Cardiac arrhythmias. In *Heart Diseases in Infancy and Childhood,* Keith J, Rowe R, and Vlad P, eds. New York: MacMillan, 1978.

34. Sinaiko A and Mirken B. Clinical pharmacology of anti-hypertensive drugs in children. *Pediatr Clin North Am* 25:137, 1978.

35. Shahar E, Barzilay Z, and Frand M. Verapamil in the treatment of paroxysmal supraventricular tachycardia in infants and children. *J Pediatr* 98:323, 1981.

36. Greco R, Musto B, Arienzo V, et al. Treatment of paroxysmal supraventricular tachycardia in infancy with digitalis, adenosine-5'-triphosphate, and verapamil: A comparative study. *Circulation* 66:504, 1982.

Respiratory Drug Therapy

Medication	Indication	Dosage/route
Caffeine	Apnea of prematurity	Loading dose: [1] 10 mg/kg (20 mg/kg caffeine citrate) PO Maintenance dose: 2.5 mg/kg/day (5 mg/kg/day caffeine citrate) PO Administer the first maintenance dose 24 hours after the loading dose.
Theophylline	Apnea of prematurity, [3] bronchopulmonary dysplasia	Loading dose: [1,4] 5.5-6.0 mg/kg IV over a minimum of 10 minutes Maintenance dose: 1 mg/kg every 8 hours or 2 mg/kg every 12 hours A low-dose regimen has been used. Loading dose: 2.5 mg/kg Maintenance dose: 2 mg/kg/day in 3 divided doses, yielding a plasma concentration of 2.8-3.9 mcg/ml
Tolazoline (Priscoline)	Persistent fetal circulation, pulmonary hypertension	Loading dose: [5,6] 0.5-2 mg/kg IV over 10 minutes IV infusion: 0.5-2 mg/kg/hour

Therapeutic range	Side effects		Comment
8-20 [1] mcg/ml; time of sample, trough level: prior to the next dose	Jitteriness* (with serum levels >50 mcg/ml)	[2]	Parenteral form not recommended. This product contains sodium benzoate, which displaces bilirubin from its protein-binding sites.
5-12 [1] mcg/ml; time of sample, trough level: prior to the next dose; peak level: 30-60 min after the dose; caffeine level should be monitored.	Gastrointestinal disturbances— abdominal distention, vomiting— tachycardia, arrhythmias,* seizure*	[2]	Multiply the dose of theophylline by a factor of 1.25 to calculate the dose of aminophylline.
N/A	Hypotension, thrombocytopenia, GI bleeding, oliguria (may be secondary to hypoxia, not drug therapy)	[6,7]	Efficacy of the drug in pulmonary hypertension is questionable.

*Toxic manifestations.

References

1. Aranda J, Grondin D, and Sasyniuk B. Pharmacologic considerations in the therapy of neonatal apnea. *Pediatr Clin North Am* 28:113, 1982.

2. Howell J, Clozel M, and Aranda J. Adverse effects of caffeine and theophylline in the newborn infant. *Semin Perinatol* 5:359, 1981.

3. Rooklin AR, Moomjian AS, Shutack JG, et al. Theophylline therapy in bronchopulmonary dysplasia. *J Pediatr* 95:882, 1979.

4. Milsap R, Krauss A, and Auld P. Efficacy of low-dose theophylline. *Semin Perinatol* 5:321, 1981.

5. Drummond WH, Gregory GA, Heyman MA, et al. The independent effects of hyperventilation, tolazoline, and dopamine on infants with persistent pulmonary hypertension. *J Pediatr* 98:603, 1981.

6. Hegyi T and Hiatt M. Tolazoline and dopamine therapy in neonatal hypoxia and pulmonary vasospasm. *Acta Paediatr Scand* 69:101, 1980.

7. Stevens DC, Schreiner RL, Bull MJ, et al. An analysis of tolazoline therapy in the critically ill neonate. *J Pediatr Surg* 15:964, 1980.

Anticonvulsant Drug Therapy

Medication	Indication	Dosage/route
Diazepam (Valium)	Status epilepticus	0.1-0.3 mg/kg IV or rectal; maximum dose, 2 mg; administer IV dose over 2-5 min [1]
Paraldehyde	Seizures not responsive to phenobarbital and phenytoin	0.15 ml/kg PO, rectal, or IM every 4-6 hours or IV infusion of a 4% solution; titrate dose to control seizures [1]
Phenobarbital	Seizures	Loading dose: 15-20 mg/kg PO, IM, or IV [6,7,8,9,10] Maintenance dose: 3-5 mg/kg/day PO, IM, or IV in 2 divided doses

Therapeutic range	Side effects		Comment
N/A	Respiratory failure, displacement of bilirubin from protein binding sites (sodium benzoate in the parenteral dosage form)	1,2	Not recommended as a first-line drug in neonates
N/A	Pneumonitis, irritation to tissues (IM, rectal), sterile abscess at site of injection, thrombosis, metabolic acidosis, pulmonary edema	3,4	Contra- 1,3,5 indicated in infants with respiratory disease. Avoid plastic containers. Use freshly prepared drug only; decomposed drug is toxic.
15-40 1,6,9 mcg/ml; time of sample, trough level: prior to the next dose	Lethargy, respiratory depression, osteomalacia with long-term therapy	11	This is drug of choice for seizures.

Medication	Indication	Dosage/route
Phenytoin	Seizures	Loading dose: 15-20 mg/kg IV [6,8] Maintenance dose: 3-8 mg/kg/day IV in 2 divided doses Administer at a rate <50 mg/min

Therapeutic range		Side effects		Comment
6-14 mcg/ml; time of sample, trough level: prior to the next dose	*9*	Hypertrichosis, gingival hyperplasia, osteomalacia with long-term therapy, skin eruptions, lymphadenopathy, hepatitis, hematologic abnormalities, folate deficiency, hyperglycemia, extrapyramidal movements,* exacerbation of the seizure disorder,* encephalopathy (chronic intoxication)*	*11*	Absorption of the drug given orally is incomplete and unreliable.

*Toxic manifestations.

References

1. Volpe J and Koenigsberger R. Neurologic disorders. In *Neonatology, Pathophysiology and Management of the Newborn,* Avery GB, ed. Philadelphia: Lippincott, 1981.

2. Langslet A, Meberg A, Breseden JE, et al. Plasma concentrations of diazepam and N-desmethyldiazepam in newborn infants after intravenous, intramuscular, rectal, and oral administration. *Acta Paediatr Scand* 67:699, 1978.

3. Holden KB and Freeman JM. Neonatal seizures and their treatment. *Clin Perinatol* 2:3, 1975.

4. Bostrom B. Paraldehyde toxicity during treatment of status epilepticus. *Am J Dis Child* 136:414, 1982.

5. Morris H. Current treatment of status epilepticus. *J Fam Prac* 13:987, 1981.

6. Painter MJ, Pippenger C, MacDonald H, et al. Phenobarbital and diphenylhydantoin levels in neonates with seizures. *J Pediatr* 92:315, 1978.

7. Lockman LA, Kriel R, Zaske D, et al. Phenobarbital dosage for control of neonatal seizures. *Neurology* 29:1445, 1979.

8. Painter MJ, Pippenger C, Wasterlain C, et al. Phenobarbital and phenytoin in neonatal seizures: Metabolism and tissue distribution. *Neurology* 31:1107, 1981.

9. Johnston MV and Freeman JH. Pharmacologic advances in seizure control. *Pediatr Clin North Am* 28:179, 1981.

10. Fischer JH, Lockman LA, Zaske D, et al. Phenobarbital maintenance dose requirements in treating neonatal seizures. *Neurology* 31:1042, 1981.

11. Penry JD and Newmark ME. The use of antiepileptic drugs. *Ann Intern Med* 90:207, 1979.

Endocrine Therapy

Medication	Indication	Dosage/route
Cortisone	Adrenal insufficiency requiring glucocorticoid replacement	0.25 mg/kg PO, every 6 hours [1,2]
Desoxycorticosterone (Percorten)	Adrenal insufficiency requiring mineralocorticoid replacement	1-2 mg IM every 12 hours [3]
Dexamethasone	Cerebral edema	Loading dose: [1] 0.2-0.5 mg Maintenance dose: 0.1 mg/kg IV every 6-8 hours
Diazoxide (Proglycem)	Hyperinsulinism	10-20 mg/kg/day [4] PO in 3 or 4 divided doses
9 × Fludrocortisone (Florinef)	Adrenal insufficiency requiring mineralocorticoid replacement	0.1-0.2 mg/day [3] PO

Side effects	Comment
Immunosuppression, hyperglycemia, sodium retention, growth suppression	Side effects occur with excess dosage.
	Monitor serum [3] electrolytes, weight, and blood pressure. Oral salt supplementation—2-3 g daily in divided doses—is needed.
Adrenal suppression; see cortisone	
Congestive heart failure, [4] hyperglycemia, increased uric acid levels	
	Monitor serum [3] electrolytes, weight, and blood pressure. Oral salt supplementation—2-3 g/day in divided doses—is needed.

Medication	Indication	Dosage/route
Glucagon	Hypoglycemia	50-100 mcg/kg IM [4] every 6-12 hours as needed
Hydrocortisone	Adrenal crisis requiring glucocorticoid replacement	Loading dose: [2,3] 50 mg IV bolus Maintenance dose: 20 mg/M^2/day in 3 divided doses
	Hypoglycemia	10 mg/kg/day in 2 divided doses
Insulin	Diabetic acidosis, glycosuria	1 unit SQ every [1,5] 4 hours; taper dose with improvement Infusion: 0.01-0.1 units/kg/hour
L-Thyroxine	Hypothyroidism	0.01-0.2 [6] mg/kg/day PO (200-300 mcg/M^2/day)
Vasopressin	Diabetes insipidus	Aqueous: 1-3 ml/day SQ in 3 divided doses Tannate in oil: 0.2 ml/dose IM every 1-3 days Nose drops: 1-2 drops at bedtime and every 4-6 hours as needed

Side effects	Comment
Rebound hypoglycemia	
See cortisone	
Hypoglycemia	Titrate dosage 5 to achieve desired glucose concentration.
Hyperthyroidism	

References

1. Avery G. *Neonatology*. Philadelphia: Lippincott, 1981.

2. Gutai JP and Migeon C. Adrenal insufficiency during the neonatal period. *Clin Perinatol* 2:163, 1975.

3. Hughes I. Congenital and acquired disorders of the adrenal cortex. *Clin Endocrinol Metab* 11:89, 1982.

4. Aynsley-Green A. Hypoglycemia in infants and children. *Clin Endocrinol Metab* 11:159, 1982.

5. Blumer JL and Blumenfeld TA. Therapeutic agents. In *Behrman's Neonatal-Perinatal Medicine,* 3rd ed, Fanaroff AA and Martin RJ, eds. St. Louis: Mosby, 1983.

6. MacGilliuray M. Thyroid dysfunction in the neonatal period. *Clin Perinatol* 2:15, 1975.

Miscellaneous Medications

Medication	Indication	Dosage/route	
Albumin	Hypovolemia	1 g/kg IV slowly	1
Belladonna	Anticholinergic agent	0.1 ml/kg/day PO in 3 or 4 divided doses	1
Chloral hydrate	Sedation	25-50 mg/kg PO or rectal	1
Cholestyramine (Questran)	Intractable diarrhea	Up to 4-8 g/day PO in 3-6 divided doses	3,4
Edrophonium (Tensilon)	Test for myasthenia gravis	0.1 ml SQ or IM	6
Heparin	Anticoagulant	100 units/kg IV every 4 hours as needed or Infusion	7
		Loading dose: 50 units/kg Maintenance dose: Small premature infant, 20 units/kg/hour; larger premature infants or full-term infants, 25 units/kg/hour	
		Increase dose by 5 units/hour to achieve desired therapeutic response.	

Side effects		Comment
Circulatory overload	*1*	
Flushing, hyperthermia, dry secretions	*2*	
Hyperchloremic acidosis, fat malabsorption, steatorrhea, intestinal obstruction, constipation	*3,4,5*	Binds other drugs
		Obtain baseline coagulation studies: APTT, PT, platelet count, fibrinogen, clotting time. *7* Adjust therapy following the clotting time or, less preferably, APTT.

Medication	Indication	Dosage/route
Kayexalate	See Polystyrene sulfonate	
Mannitol	Cerebral edema	0.25-0.5 g/kg [2] IV over 30-60 minutes; repeat every 8-12 hours as needed
Meperidine	Pain	1 mg/kg PO or IM [2] every 4-6 hours as needed
Morphine sulfate	Pain	0.1 mg/kg IV [6] every 4-6 hours as needed
Naloxone (Narcan)	Reversal of narcotic depression	0.01 mg/kg/dose [8] IV or IM; repeat as needed
Neostigmine	Test for myasthenia gravis	0.04 mg/kg IM [2]
Pancuronium bromide (Pavulon)	Paralysis	0-7 days: [9] 0.03 mg/kg IV 1-2 weeks: 0.06 mg/kg IV 2-4 weeks: 0.09 mg/kg IV
Polystyrene sulfonate (Kayexalate)	Hyperkalemia	0.5-1 g/kg PO or [1] as a sorbitol 25% enema every 6 hours as needed

Side effects		Comment
Circulatory overload, rebound edema	2	
CNS depression, theoretical risk of seizures from accumulation of normeperidine		
CNS depression		
		Infants addicted to narcotics will go through drug withdrawal.
Cardiac arrhythmias	2	Use atropine as antidote.
		Conditions and medications 7 potentiating or prolonging drug activity: hypokalemia, acidosis, administration of magnesium sulfate, decreased renal function, aminoglycosides, local anesthetics, quinidine
		Monitor serum potassium.

Medication	Indication	Dosage/route
Protamine	Heparin overdose	1 mg IV for each [1,2] 100 units of heparin administered in the last 4 hours
Tubocurarine (Curare)	Paralysis	0-7 days: [9] 0.2 mg/kg IV 1-2 weeks: 0.3 mg/kg IV 2-4 weeks: 0.4 mg/kg IV

Side effects	Comment
Hypotension	See pancuronium bromide. 7

References

1. Blumer JL and Blumenfeld TA. Therapeutic agents. In *Behrman's Neonatal-Perinatal Medicine,* 3rd ed, Fanaroff AA and Martin RJ, eds. St. Louis: Mosby, 1983.

2. Avery G. *Neonatology.* Philadelphia: Lippincott, 1981.

3. Nagaraj HS, Cook L, Canty TG, et al. Oral cholestyramine and paregoric therapy for intractable diarrhea following surgical correction of catastrophic disease of the GI tract in neonates. *J Pediatr Surg* 11:795, 1976.

4. Tamer MA, Santora TR, and Sandberg DH. Cholestyramine therapy for intractable diarrhea. *Pediatrics* 53:217, 1974.

5. Nicolopoulos D. Combined treatment of neonatal jaundice with cholestyramine and phototherapy. *J Pediatr* 93:684, 1978.

6. Cloherty J and Stark A, eds. *Manual of Neonatal Care.* Boston: Little, Brown, 1980.

7. McDonald M and Hathaway W. Anticoagulant therapy by continuous heparinization in newborn and older infants. *J Pediatr* 101:451, 1982.

8. American Academy of Pediatrics, Committee on Drugs. Naloxone use in newborns. *Pediatrics* 65:667, 1980.

9. Nugent S, Laravuso R, and Rogers H. Pharmacology and use of muscle relaxants in infants and children. *J Pediatr* 94:481, 1979.

Drug Withdrawal

SIGNS AND SYMPTOMS[1,2,3]

Tremor	Marked sucking
Hyperactivity	Poor feeding
Irritability	Nasal stuffiness
Hypertonicity	Sneezing
Persistent crying	Yawning
Tachypnea	Sweating
>60 breaths/minute	Seizures
Hyperpyrexia	Sleep disturbances
Vomiting, diarrhea	

ONSET OF SYMPTOMS

• Heroin: 24-48 hours.[1,2]

• Methadone: Usual onset of symptoms occurs within 72 hours, but may occur up to two weeks after birth.[2,3]

• Barbiturate: Symptoms begin at a median of 7 days (range 2-14 days). Delayed onset may be due to the slow metabolism and elimination of phenobarbital in the newborn.

• Diazepam (Valium): 24 hours, according to three case reports.[4]

• Codeine, pentazocine (Talwin), and propoxyphene have been reported to cause withdrawal symptoms.

MANAGEMENT

From 10 to 30% of infants with withdrawal symptoms can be managed by swaddling, placement in a quiet environment, and small frequent feedings. Infants who feed poorly, cry continuously, or show signs of irritability and tremor should be sedated.[2,3]

Medications: Tincture of opium USP (laudanum) is a 10% solution that contains 1% morphine. Dilute 25-fold to yield a concentration of morphine equivalent to that of paregoric (0.4% opium, 0.04% morphine.)[2] The dose is 0.05 ml/kg every 3 or 4 hours. This dose may be increased by 0.05 ml every 4 hours until a clinical response is achieved. Once an adequate dose is attained, the dose may be tapered by 10% daily.[5] Side effects include sedation and constipation.

Paregoric is as effective as tincture of opium, but has several disadvantages. Paregoric is a compound containing several ingredients—opium tincture, anise oil, benzoic acid, camphor, glycerine, alcohol—that are not therapeutically useful and may even be harmful:

• Benzoic acid administered parenterally displaces bilirubin from its albumin binding sites. Although oral administration has not been shown to displace bilirubin, there is a theoretical risk.[2]

• Camphor is a central nervous system stimulant that is rapidly absorbed and slowly excreted in the newborn.[2]

• Tincture of opium seems to be preferable, if a narcotic is to be administered. The dose and side effects of paregoric are the same as with tincture of opium.

Phenobarbital is effective in controlling symptoms of withdrawal, with the exception of gastrointestinal manifestations. The initial dose of phenobarbital is 20 mg/kg over 24 hours followed by a maintenance dose of 4-6 mg/kg/day in 2 divided doses.[1] The side effects include poor sucking and sedation.

Chlorpromazine is administered at a dose of 0.7-0.8 mg/kg every 6 hours by IM injection. The drug may be given by mouth once the patient is stable.[3] The disadvantages of this medication include the risks of hypotension and hypothermia and a prolonged excretion time in the newborn.

Diazepam has no advantage over the other medications and is associated with several problems. The parenteral formulation of diazepam contains sodium benzoate, which may displace bilirubin from its albumin binding sites, increasing the risk of kernicterus. Bradycardia and respiratory depression have occurred after intravenous administration.[3] Newborns have a limited capacity to excrete diazepam. Persistent levels of the drug in blood and tissues permit a rapid decrease in dosage and early discharge from the nursery, but the risk of recurrence of withdrawal symptoms at home is a serious disadvantage. The suggested dose of diazepam is 1-2 mg IM every 12 hours until symptoms are controlled. The dose is then decreased by half and administered every 12 hours. The dose is lowered until 0.5 mg is reached, and then the drug is discontinued.[3,5]

Clonidine (Catapres) has been reported to be effective in the management of narcotic withdrawal symptoms in the newborn.[6] Initially, the infant was given a dose of 0.5-1 mcg/kg orally, and observed. Twenty-four hours later a dose of 3-4 mcg/kg/day was administered orally in 4 divided doses. No adverse reactions were reported, although there is a risk of hypotension when using clonidine. Further studies are needed to determine the safety and efficacy of this medication prior to its routine use in newborns with withdrawal symptoms.[5]

References

1. Rosen TS. Infants of addicted mothers. In *Behrman's Neonatal-Perinatal Medicine,* 3rd ed, Fanaroff AA and Martin RJ, eds. St. Louis: Mosby, 1983.

2. Neumann L and Cohen S. The neonatal narcotic withdrawal syndrome. *Clin Perinatol* 2:99, 1975.

3. Sweet A. Narcotic withdrawal syndrome in the newborn. *Pediatr Rev* 3:285, 1982.

4. Rementeria J and Bhatt K. Withdrawal symptoms in neonates from intrauterine exposure to diazepam. *J Pediatr* 99:123, 1977.

5. Cloherty J. Drug withdrawal. In *Manual of Neonatal Care,* Cloherty J and Stark A, eds. Boston: Little, Brown, 1980.

6. Hoder EL, Leckman JF, Ehrenkranz R, et al. Clonidine in neonatal narcotic-abstinence syndrome. *N Engl J Med* 305:1284, 1981.

SECTION 11

Nutritional Requirements

Nutrient	Recommended daily intake	Comment
Calories	100-120 cal/kg [1]	Caloric requirements [2] may be increased with fever, cold, stress, systemic illness, and increased activity. Caloric requirements are decreased—80-120 cal/kg—in infants fed parenterally.
Protein	2.5-3 g/kg, [2,4,5] 7-16% of total caloric intake	**Essential amino acids** [2,4,5] Threonine — Valine Leucine — Lysine Isoleucine — Methionine Phenylalanine — Tryptophan Histidine (for infants) Tyrosine* Cystine* Taurine*
Carbohydrates	11-16 g/kg, [3] 35-50% of the total caloric intake	
Fat	2-3 g/kg, [3] 40-50% of total caloric intake	Linoleic acid is an essential fatty acid. Two to 3% of the infant's total caloric intake should be in the form of linoleic acid to prevent essential fatty acid deficiency. Infants receiving medium-chain triglycerides as their only source of fat may develop essential fatty acid deficiency.

*Possibly needed by premature infants.

MINERALS[1,3,6,7]

Nutrient	Recommended daily intake	Comment
Sodium	2-3 mEq/kg	Premature infants may require up to 8-10 mEq/kg/day.
Potassium	2-3 mEq/kg	Premature infants may require up to 8-10 mEq/kg/day.
Chloride	2 mEq/kg	
Calcium	20-40 mg/kg; premature infants, 150-200 mg/kg	Oral calcium supplementation— calcium gluconate 9 mg Ca/ml or calcium glubionate 23 mg Ca/ml— may be needed in premature infants.
Phosphorus	20-40 mg/kg	Quantity to achieve a calcium-to-phosphorus ratio of 2:1 in premature infants.
Magnesium	3-4 mg/kg	
Iron	Premature infants, 2 mg/kg/ day; full-term infants, 1 mg/kg/day [6]	
Fluoride	0.5 mg/day	Not needed if water contains fluoride.

VITAMINS[8]

Nutrient	Recommended daily intake	
	Premature	Full term
Vitamin A	500 IU	250 IU
Vitamin D	400-600 IU	40-100 IU
Vitamin E	30 IU Administer 25 IU vitamin E as prophylaxis for infants less than 2 kg.	4 IU
Vitamin K	15 mcg Administer 0.5-1 mg/kg vitamin K IM at birth to prevent hemorrhagic disease of the newborn.	4 mcg
Vitamin C	60 mg	8 mg
Thiamine (B_1)	0.2 mg	0.04 mg

| Nutrient | Recommended daily intake | |
	Premature	Full term
Riboflavin (B_2)	0.4 mg	0.06 mg
Pyridoxine (B_6)	0.4 mg	0.035 mg
Niacin	5 mg	4 mcg
Vitamin B_{12}	1.5 mcg	0.15 mcg
Pantothenic acid	2 mg	1.5 mcg
Folic acid	6 mg	0.3 mg
Biotin	12 mcg	7 mcg

COW'S MILK, HUMAN MILK, AND FORMULAS[9, 10, 11]

Formula	Caloric content per 100 ml	Protein quantity g/100 ml whey/casein	Carbohydrate quantity g/100 ml—type	Fat quantity g/100 ml—type
Cow's milk, whole	67	3.4 18/82	4.8—lactose	3.7—butterfat
Human milk, mature	73	1.1 60/40	7.0—lactose	4.5—human milk fat
Enfamil 20 With Iron	67	1.5 60/40	7.0—lactose	3.8—soy and coconut oils
Similac PM 60/40	68	1.58 60/40	6.88—lactose	3.7—coconut and corn oils
Similac With Iron 20	68	1.55 18/82	7.2—lactose	3.6—soy and coconut oils
Similac With Iron 24	81	2.2 18/82	8.5—lactose	4.3—soy and coconut oils
Similac With Whey 20	68	1.55 60/40	7.2—lactose	3.6—soy and coconut oils

Na mEq/L	K mEq/L	Ca mg/L P mg/L ratio	Iron mg/L	Osmolarity mosm/L	Approximate renal solute load mosm/L
22	40	1230/960 1.3:1	0.5	260	230
8.5	15	330/150 2:1	1.5	270	75
9	18	466/317 1.5:1	1.0 (12)	250	
7	15	400/200 2:1	2.6	240	92
11	20	510/390 1.3:1	1.5 (12)	260	108
16	28	730/560 1.3:1	1.8 (15)	320	152
10	19	400/300 1.3:1	1.8 (15)	270	104

Formula	Caloric content per 100 ml	Protein quantity g/100 ml whey/casein	Carbohydrate quantity g/100 ml—type	Fat quantity g/100 ml—type
Similac 24 LBW	81	2.2 18/82	8.5—lactose and corn syrup solids	4.5—medium-chain tri-glycerides, coconut and soy oils
SMA Lo-Iron 20	68	1.5 60/40	7.2—lactose	3.6—oleo, coconut, safflower, and soy oils
SMA 24	81	1.8 60/40	8.6—lactose	4.3—oleo, coconut, safflower, and soy oils

Na mEq/L	K mEq/L	Ca mg/L P mg/L ratio	Iron mg/L	Osmolarity mosm/L	Approximate renal solute load mosm/L
16	31	730/560 1.3:1	3.0	260	160
6	14	440/330 1.3:1	12.7 (1.5)	270	90
8	17	530/390 1.35/1	15.0	320	109

FORMULAS FOR PREMATURE INFANTS[9, 10]

Formula	Caloric content per 100 ml	Protein quantity g/100 ml whey/casein	Carbohydrate quantity g/100 ml—type	Fat quantity g/100 ml—type
Enfamil Premature Formula	81	2.4 60/40	8.9—lactose	4.1—medium-chain tri-glycerides, corn and coconut oils
"Preemie" SMA	81	2.0 60/40	8.6—lactose and corn syrup solids	4.4—medium-chain tri-glycerides, coconut, oleic, oleo, and soy oils
Similac Special Care 20	68	1.8 60/40	7.2—lactose and corn syrup solids	3.7—medium-chain tri-glycerides, corn and coconut oils
Similac Special Care 24	81	2.2 60/40	8.6—lactose and corn syrup solids	4.4—medium-chain tri-glycerides, corn and coconut oils

Na mEq/L	K mEq/L	Ca mg/L P mg/L ratio	Iron mg/L	Osmolarity mosm/L	Approximate renal solute load mosm/L
14	23	950/480 2:1	1.3	270	180
14	19	750/400 1.8:1	3.0	240	128
13	21	1200/600 2:1	2.5	220	122
15	26	1440/720 2:1	3.0	260	147

SPECIAL DIET FORMULAS[9, 10]

Formula	Caloric content per 100 ml	Protein quantity g/100 ml whey/casein	Carbohydrate quantity g/100 ml—source	Fat quantity g/100 ml— source	Na mEq/L
Isomil 20	68	2.0—soy protein	6.8—corn syrup solids and sucrose	3.6—soy and coconut oils	13
Isomil SF 20	68	2.0—soy protein	6.8— glucose polymers	3.6—soy and coconut oils	13
Lofenalac	68	2.2— processed casein hydrolysate	8.8—corn syrup solids	2.7— corn oil	8
Nursoy	68	2.1—soy protein	6.9—sucrose	3.6—oleo, coconut, safflower, and soy oils	9
Nutramigen	68	2.2—casein hydrolysate	8.8—sucrose, tapioca, starch	2.6— corn oil	14

K mEq/L	Ca mg/L P mg/L ratio	Iron mg/L	Osmolarity mosm/L	Approximate solute load renal/GI mosm/L	Use
18	700/500 1.4:1	12	230	126	Lactose or cow's protein intolerance; caution: Long-term use in low-birth-weight infants is not recommended without calcium supplementation.
18	700/500 1.4:1	12	140	130/407	Lactose, sucrose, and/or cow's milk intolerance; caution: See Isomil 20
30	634/475 1.3:1	12.6	320	140/ —	Low phenylalanine diet
19	630/440 1.3:1	12.7			Lactose and/or cow's milk intolerance; caution: See Isomil 20
17	630/473 1.3:1	13	431	130/397	Infants sensitive to intact proteins of milk, lactose intolerance, and galactosemia; caution: high GI solute load

Formula	Caloric content per 100 ml	Protein quantity g/100 ml whey/casein	Carbohydrate quantity g/100 ml—source	Fat quantity g/100 ml— source	Na mEq/L
Portagen	68	2.4—casein	7.8—sucrose and corn syrup solids	3.2— medium- chain tri- glycerides and corn oil	14
Pregestimil	68	2.0—casein hydrolysate	9.1—corn syrup solids, tapioca, starch	2.7— medium- chain tri- glycerides and corn oil	14
Prosobee	68	2.0—soy protein	6.9—corn syrup solids	3.6—soy oil and coconut oil	13

K mEq/L	Ca mg/L P mg/L ratio	Iron mg/L	Osmolarity mosm/L	Approximate solute load renal/GI mosm/L	Use
21	600/450 1.3:1	13	136	150/211	Fat malabsorption
17	634/422 1.5:1	12	311	130/297	Infants with severe food allergies, sensitivity to intact proteins, disaccharidase deficiency, fat malabsorption; caution: high GI solute load
21	634/502	13	180	127/233	Cow's protein and/or lactose intolerance; caution: See Isomil 20

PARENTERAL NUTRITION

GENERAL INDICATIONS

- Low-birth-weight infants receiving inadequate calories by the oral route.[12]
- Gastrointestinal disorders, including effects of surgery, chronic diarrhea, and necrotizing enterocolitis.
- Severe respiratory distress.

CENTRAL VENOUS ALIMENTATION[13,14,15]

- Indicated in infants requiring hypertonic dextrose solutions to supply calories. The introduction of a fat preparation for parenteral administration has provided an alternative source of calories.

- Complications include bacteremia, septicemia, fungemia, pleural effusion, pulmonary emboli, hemorrhage, perforation of the central veins, and superior vena cava thrombophlebitis and thrombosis.
- Monitoring parameters (infection): CBC (weekly), temperature (daily), blood cultures.

SUGGESTED DISTRIBUTION OF CALORIES[4]

- Protein 10-15%
- Fat 45-50%
- Carbohydrate to make necessary calories.

PARENTERAL NUTRITION THERAPEUTIC PLAN

Nutrient	Source	Quantity	
Fluid	Oral and parenteral intake	130-140 ml/kg/day; initial rate in low-birth-weight infants is 40-60 ml/kg/day. Increase rate slowly as tolerated. *Note: Premature infants may have increased fluid requirements.*	13
Calories	Carbohydrates and fat	90-120 cal/kg/day	16
Protein	Crystalline amino acid solutions	2-3 g/kg/day	13

Complications	Monitoring parameters	

Complications	Parameter	Frequency
DEHYDRATION *16*		*8,9,11,12,13,14*
Conditions requiring greater fluid intake: prematurity, radiant heat (with phototherapy or radiant warmers), increased activity, cold stress, fever, GI losses	Volume of infusate	Daily
	Oral intake	Daily
	Urinary output	Daily
	Urine specific gravity or osmolarity	With each voiding
OVERHYDRATION	Weight	Daily
Conditions requiring decreased fluid intake: renal failure, congestive heart failure, meningitis	Skin turgor	Daily
	Anterior fontanelle	Daily
	Plasma sodium	Minimum 2x/week
	Plasma osmolarity	Daily
	BUN	3x/week
	Hematocrit	2-3x/week
	Creatinine	Weekly
	Temperature	Daily
	Weight	Daily *12, 13*
	Length	Weekly
	Head circumference	Weekly
Azotemia, hyperammonemia, *13* metabolic acidosis (rare with current formulations), possible hepatotoxicity	BUN	2-3x/week *12, 13*
	Serum albumin	Weekly
	Blood NH_3	2-3x/week
	Acid-base status	3x/week
	Liver function tests	Weekly

PARENTERAL NUTRITION PLAN *continued*

Nutrient	Source	Quantity
Carbohydrate	Dextrose	11-16 g/kg/day, peripherally; greater concentrations may be infused through a central line. *3*
Fat	Intralipid 10% 20% Liposyn 10% 20%	1-4 g/kg/day *13*
Sodium	Sodium chloride	2-4 mEq/day *3, 16*
Potassium	Potassium chloride and/or potassium phosphate	2-3 mEq/day *3, 16*
Chloride	Sodium chloride, potassium chloride	2-3 mEq/day *3*

Complications	Monitoring parameters	
Hyperglycemia 24-48 hours 13 after increasing glucose concentration, sepsis, hypoglycemia (discontinue glucose abruptly)	Blood glucose Urine glucose	Minimum daily 3 Each void for 1 week, then every shift
Alteration of pulmonary 13 function, displacement of bilirubin from protein binding sites, hypercholesterolemia, hypertriglyceridemia, overloading syndrome—fat load exceeds the infant's ability to clear it—thrombocytopenia, possible hepatotoxicity	Visual inspection of plasma for turbidity Serum-free fatty acids Serum triglyceride and cholesterol Platelets Liver function tests—bilirubin Urine ketones	Daily 12, 13 prior to fat infusion Weekly Weekly Weekly Weekly Each void for 1 week, then every shift
Hypernatremia, hyponatremia	Serum sodium	3x/week 12, 13 when stable
Hyperkalemia, hypokalemia	Serum potassium	3x/week 12, 13 when stable
Hyperchloremic metabolic acidosis	Blood acid-base balance	3x/week 12, 13

Nutrient	Source	Quantity	
Calcium	Calcium gluconate	1-2 mEq/kg/day (20-40 mg/kg/day) *Note: Premature infants require an additional supplement—150-200 mg/kg/day enterally when tolerated.*	*3,16*
Phosphorus	Potassium phosphate	2 mM/kg/day	
Magnesium	Magnesium sulfate	0.25-0.5 mEq/kg	*13*
Zinc	Zinc sulfate	300 mcg/kg for premature infants 100 mcg/kg for full-term infants	*18*
Copper Chromium Manganese	Cupric sulfate	20 mcg/kg 0.14-0.2 mcg/kg 2-10 mcg/kg	*18* *18* *18*

Complications	Monitoring parameters		
Hypercalcemia, hypocalcemia	Serum calcium Alkaline phosphatase	Weekly 2x/month	*3*
Hyperphosphatemia, hypophosphatemia	Serum phosphorus	Weekly	*12, 13*
Hypermagnesemia, hypomagnesemia (both rare)	Serum magnesium	Weekly	*12, 13*

PARENTERAL NUTRITION PLAN *continued*

Nutrient	Source	Quantity	
Vitamins	Multivitamins	Quantity/1 ml	
		Vitamin A	2000 IU
		Vitamin B	200 IU
		Vitamin E	1 IU
		Thiamine	10 mg
		Riboflavin	2 mg
		Pyridoxine	3 mg
		Niacin	20 mg
		Vitamin C	100 mg
		Dexpanthenol	5 mg
	Folic acid	50 mcg/day	*13*
	Vitamin B$_{12}$	5 mcg/day	*13*
	Vitamin K	0.5-1 mg/kg IM weekly	*3*

Complications	Monitoring parameters	
Vitamin D deficiency *17* (rickets), vitamin E deficiency (hemolytic anemia) *Note: Premature infants require 30 IU of vitamin E to prevent hemolytic anemia*	Alkaline phosphatase	2x/month
	Hemoglobin	2x/week
	Hematocrit	2x/week

References

1. Reena D. Infant nutrition. *Clin Perinatol* 2:383, 1975.

2. Nelson W, ed. *Textbook of Pediatrics.* Philadelphia: Saunders, 1979.

3. Cox M and Thrift M. Nutrition. In *Manual of Neonatal Care,* Cloherty J and Stark A, eds. Boston: Little, Brown, 1980.

4. Malloy MH and Gaull G. Enteral protein and amino acid nutrition in preterm infants. *Semin Perinatol* 3:315, 1979.

5. Morrow G. Protein and infant formulas. *Semin Perinatol* 3:321, 1979.

6. Avery G. *Neonatology.* Philadelphia: Lippincott, 1981.

7. Oski F. Nutritional anemias. *Semin Perinatol* 3:381, 1979.

8. Suskind RM, ed. *Textbook of Pediatric Nutrition.* New York: Raven, 1981.

9. Product Literature. Evansville, Ind: Mead, Johnson, and Company, 1981.

10. Product Literature. Columbus, Ohio: Ross, 1982.

11. Fleischman A and Finberg L. Breast milk for term and premature infants: Optimal nutrition? *Semin Perinatol* 3:397, 1979.

12. Heird WC and Anderson TL. Nutritional requirements and methods of feeding low-birth-weight infants. In *Current Problems in Pediatrics,* Gluck L, ed. Chicago: Year Book, 1977.

13. Kerner J and Sunshine P. Parenteral alimentation. *Semin Perinatol* 3:417, 1979.

14. Coran A. Parenteral nutrition in infants and children. *Surg Clin North Am* 61:1089, 1981.

15. Dweck HS. Feeding the prematurely born infant. *Clin Perinatol* 2:183, 1975.

16. Lorch V and Lay SA. Parenteral alimentation in the neonate. *Pediatr Clin North Am* 24:547, 1977.

17. Ehrenkranz R. Vitamin E and the neonate. *Am J Dis Child* 134:1157, 1980.

18. American Medical Association Department of Foods and Nutrition. Guidelines for essential trace element preparations for parenteral use. *JAMA* 241: 2051, 1979.

INDEX

premature ventricular
  contractions, 57
sinus, 59
supraventricular, 56, 64, 66
ventricular, 59, 62, 63, 65, 68
Asphyxia, perinatal, 61
Aspirin, and nursing infant,
  19
Asystole, 58, 65, 67, 68
Atropine
  dosage, 54, 68
  indications, 54, 57, 65, 68, 93
  neonate, in, 54-55, 68
  side effects, 55
AV-block, 54, 57, 67

B
Barbiturates
  lactation, and, 16
  nursing infant, and, 19
  withdrawal, 98
Belladonna, 90-91
Benzodiazepines, and
  nursing infant, 17
Benzoic acid, 99
Beta-blockers, 67
Bile
  acids, impaired synthesis, 25
  cholestasis, 35, 63
Bilirubin
  competition with, 27
  displacement, 27, 61, 75, 79,
    99, 100, 123
  elevated, 27, 41
  hyperbilirubinemia, 6, 45
  test, 123
Bioavailability, drug, 24-26, 60
Bleeding. *See* Hemorrhage/
  bleeding

Bleeding time, 41
Blood
  ammonia in, 121
  azotemia, 121
  bacteremia, 119
  drug in, 18, 29
  dyscrasias, 18, 20, 81
  eosinophilia, 41
  glucose, 123. *See also*
    Hyperglycemia;
    Hypoglycemia
  hemoperfusion, 57
  methemoglobinemia, 20
  plasma, monitoring,
    121, 123
  septicemia, 119
Blood flow
  regional, 25, 26
  renal, 31, 58
Blood pressure, 85, 87
Bone marrow
  depression, 17
  megaloblastosis, 47
  suppression, 35, 43, 45, 63
Bradycardia
  side effect, as, 3, 7, 20, 55,
    57, 65, 67, 100
  treatment of, 54, 58, 60,
    65, 68
Bromides, and nursing infant,
  17
Bromocriptine (Parlodel), and
  lactation, 16

C
Caffeine
  dosage, 74
  indications, 74
  interactions, 57

Propoxyphene, 98
Propranolol (Inderal)
  dosage, 64
  fetus/neonate, and, 7
  indications, 57, 64
  neonate, in, 64-65
  nursing infant, and, 20
  side effects, 65
Propylthiouracil
  fetus/neonate, and, 11
  nursing infant, and, 19
Protamine, 94
Protein
  amino acids, 104, 115, 120
  binding, 26, 27
  breast milk, in, 20, 108
  calories, percentage of,
    104, 119
  cow's milk, in, 108
  formulas, in, 108, 110, 112,
    114, 116
  low phenylalanine diet,
    115
  monitoring, 121
  parenteral nutrition, in,
    120-121
  requirements, 104
  sensitivity to, 115, 117
  urine, in, 55
Psychotherapeutic drugs, 9-10
Pulmonary wedge pressure,
  59
Pyridoxine, and lactation, 16
Pyrimethamine (Daraprim),
  6, 42-43

Q
Quinidine, 57, 64-65, 93
Quinine, 6

R
Radiopharmaceuticals, in
  nursing, 18
Renal solute load, 109, 111,
  113, 115, 117
Reserpine
  lactation, and, 16
  nursing infant, and, 20
Respiratory arrest, 63
Respiratory depression, 2, 7,
  53, 79, 100
Respiratory distress, 118
Respiratory drug therapy,
  73-76
Respiratory failure, 79
Rifampin (Rifadin,
  Rimactane), 6, 25,
  44-45

S
Salicylates
  fetus/neonate, and, 2
  half-life, 27
Sedation, 10, 17, 19, 20, 90,
  98, 99
Seizures/convulsions
  nursing infant, in, 17, 19
  side effect, as, 3, 7, 17, 19,
    28, 39, 43, 53, 63, 65, 75,
    81, 93
  status epilepticus, 78
  treatment for, 78, 79, 80
  withdrawal, in, 98
Shock, 58, 60
Side effects, drug, 91, 93, 95,
  99, 100
  anticonvulsants, 79, 81
  antimicrobials, 35, 37, 39,
    41, 43, 45, 47